Stop Eating Junk!

In 5 Minutes A Day
For 21 Days
Let Your Unconscious Mind
Do The Work

WITHDRAWN

Steve Murray CHt.

First Printing
———————————

Body & Mind Productions

Stop Eating Junk!
In 5 Minutes a Day For 21 Days
Let Your Unconscious Mind Do The Work

Published by
Body & Mind Productions
820 Bow Creek Lane Las Vegas, NV 89134
Website: www.stopeatjunk.com
Email: bodymindheal@aol.com
© Copyright 2004 by Steve Murray
All Rights reserved

First Printing June 2004

Library of Congress Cataloging-in-Publication Data
Murray, Steve
Stop Eating Junk! In 5 Minutes a Day For 21 Days
Let Your Unconscious Mind Do The Work
/ Murray, Steve – 1st ed.
Library of Congress Control Number 2003096335
ISBN # 0-9742569-2-7
Includes bibliographical references and index.
1. Weight Loss 2. Diet 3. Health

Cover design: Alan Berrelleza, armb-design@cox.net
Type design and production: Alan Berrelleza
Copy Editor: Carol L. Craig

Printed in U.S.A.

By
Steve Murray

VIDEOS & DVDS

Preparing Mentally & Emotionally
For Cancer Surgery
A Guided Imagery Program

Preparing Mentally & Emotionally
For Cancer Chemotherapy
A Guided Imagery Program

Preparing Mentally & Emotionally
For Cancer Radiation
A Guided Imagery Program

Preparing Mentally & Emotionally
For Cancer Recovery
A Guided Imagery Program

Dissolving & Destroying Cancer Cells
A Guided Imagery Program

Pain Relief Subliminal Program
Let Your Unconscious Mind Do It!

Fear & Stress Relief Subliminal Program
Let Your Unconscious
Mind Do The Work!

30-Day Subliminal Weight Loss Program
Let Your Unconscious
Mind Do The Work!

30-Day Subliminal Stop Smoking
Program Let Your Unconscious
Mind Do The Work!

Reiki Master Attunement
Become A Reiki Master

Reiki 1st Level Attunement
Give Healing Energy To Yourself
and Others

Reiki Healing Attunement
Heal Emotional-Mental-Physical-
Spiritual Issues

Reiki 2nd Level Attunement
Learn and Use the Reiki Sacred Symbols

BOOKS

Cancer Guided Imagery Program
For Radiation, Chemotherapy, Surgery,
And Recovery

Stop Eating Junk!
In 5 Minutes A Day for 21 Days

Reiki The Ultimate Guide
Learn Sacred Symbols and Attunements
Plus Reiki Secrets You Should Know

Disclaimer

This book is sold with the understanding and intent that the publishers and author are not engaged in giving medical advice. Because of the nature of the Food Feelings Program each individual will have his or her own results with the program.

Dedication

To Shelly Stockwell

Foreword

The Food Feelings Program is a very powerful tool for weight loss. My challenge was to write a book that made the program simple to understand, with easy, straightforward instructions. I feel I have succeeded in accomplishing that and now the program is available to everyone.

If you have any questions, feel free to contact me through the publisher, or through my web site www.stopeatjunk.com

Steve Murray

Contents

Foreword

The more you eat,

the less flavor;

the less you eat,

the more flavor.

~Chinese Proverb

Chapter 1

Food Feelings Program

How would you like to reduce or even eliminate specific junk foods, or any type of food that you feel is problematic to your health or diet, and by doing so, lose weight and help prevent future health problems? Those who crave certain junk foods know that this is easier said than done. Or is it?

This book is about a fun and innovative process called the Food Feelings Program, which will show you an easy way to eliminate junk foods in your diet.

The program is personalized. You select the junk food(s) you would like to cut back on or eliminate from your diet. It can be just one food or as many as you like. Simply follow the five-minutes-per-day, 21-day program for each food you select, and then let your unconscious mind do the work. It's that simple.

Anyone can achieve success with this method. Of course, as is the case with any program, you must follow the instructions for results. You will achieve varying degrees of success with the Food Feelings Program, which is dependent on a few variables that will be explained later.

There is no special will power, pill, diet, or exercise required in order for the program to work. It can be used in conjunction with any other weight loss program you may be currently using, such as Weight Watchers, the Atkins Diet, the Hollywood Diet, or any exercise regimen. Or you can simply implement the Food Feelings Program by itself.

Even though the program does not require special diet or exercise, you will find that when you stop eating the unhealthy foods you once craved and weight loss occurs, you will feel better and have more energy to exercise and participate in other activities. Eating in a healthy manner will come more naturally as a result.

Now, before you let the words "food feelings" worry you, please understand that I am not referring to deep-rooted guilt associated with certain foods, which you might have heard of, or read about, in various psychology articles. Nor am I talking about emotions such as anger, fear, or sadness. Not only are the food feelings I am talking about different than those I just described, you will find the "feelings" in the Food Feelings Program comfortable and even fun to work with.

The program does not require an in-depth examination or a release of emotions or feelings you may or may not have connected with junk food. Many people become confused between the meanings of emotions and feelings because they can overlap. I will explain the difference in the next chapter.

Food feelings are likely not what you expect. They are a combination of different experiences, which can include emotions, feelings, and internal senses, and are unique to each person.

Food feelings are what you experience in your body right before you eat a food you like or crave. These are the same types of feelings that prevent you from eating a food you dislike. They usually happen rapidly and are felt in different locations throughout the body. Most people are completely unaware of them because they occur at the unconscious level. However, you can be made aware of these feelings, as you will learn in this book. That is the very essence of this program: becoming aware of these food feelings, and then changing them for your benefit.

I developed this program over the years by modifying and combining several well-known and not-so-well-known healing modalities and behavior techniques. Moreover, I have successfully used the program with my clients in one-on-one sessions. I have simplified the program for this book so it is easier to understand and follow. You can now do it alone and the program will be just as effective.

Three Elements

Once you have chosen the junk foods you want to reduce or eliminate altogether, you need three key elements to make the program successful:

- You need to be conscious of the food feelings of these particular junk foods.

- You need to know where the food feelings are located in your body.

- You need to move the food feelings to different locations in the body. This will result in losing the desire for these junk foods.

Initially, this process might seem baffling and challenging, but once you learn the program, it will become second nature to you. As mentioned before, I have made it a point to make the program simple to understand and implement. Once you learn it, you can use the program anytime you wish to rid yourself of a craving for a troublesome junk food.

Reasons, Explanations, and Theories

There are many reasons, explanations, and theories about why the Food Feelings Program works. They can be found in psychology and

18

science books, as well as in proven healing techniques. Explanations can also be found in the countless studies of the unconscious mind—on how it functions and why it works. I could write several in-depth books on this topic alone.

I have found, however, that the majority of people only want or need a brief overview on how and why the Food Feelings Program works before starting the program. Some people do not even care why the program works; only that it does. The overview in the next few chapters should satisfy both of the aforementioned groups.

At times I am amazed by the success of this program. Some of the reasons behind its effectiveness fall into a gray area and cannot be fully explained. So I am asking you to keep an open mind and to take a leap of faith when you utilize this program. You have nothing to lose except the desires and cravings that you have for junk foods you want to stop eating.

Pause right now and think of just one or two foods you would like to reduce or eliminate from your day-to-day eating habits. Do you know how many calories would be removed from your diet? How much weight do you think you could lose in one month, three months, six months, or a year? You will be surprised to find the answers to these and more questions as you continue reading.

Eat little, sleep sound.

~Author Unknown

Chapter 2

Food Feelings

Let's define a food feeling. It can be a feeling, an emotion, a sensation, a taste or a combination of these, and it is linked to, or associated with foods you like or dislike in your unconscious mind.

Food feelings are experienced before you eat a food, and can continue while eating. They will motivate you to either eat or avoid a food. Every person's food feelings are different and unique to each food.

How Food Feelings Are Created

In our society, we come in contact with many foods and receive plenty to eat, so a person develops many food feelings over a lifetime. If we did not have these feelings, it would be easy to eat in a healthy manner.

The feeling usually developed from your personal circumstances when you first came in contact with a food. After a period of time, the feeling was imbedded and experienced in the unconscious mind and you are now consciously unaware of this.

The food feeling can change over time, but as a rule it will stay the same once it is established, unless it is consciously changed, which you will learn how to do.

You have a food feeling for every food you have tasted, smelled, seen, and eaten in your lifetime. This feeling can be evoked by thinking of the food, hearing its name, smelling it, seeing it or eating it. Food feelings are located in various areas throughout your body, and you can locate them once you know how.

Feelings and Emotions
As I mentioned before, people are sometimes confused between the definitions of feelings and emotions. Since a food feeling can include one or the other, I will provide a definition and explanation of both.

Feelings are what we sense or experience in any part of our body, internally or externally. Random House Unabridged Dictionary has several definitions for feelings. Here are the two that most relate to a food feeling:

- Physical sensation not connected with sight,

hearing, taste or smell.

• The general state of consciousness considered independently of particular sensations and thoughts.

As we all know, feelings can be caused by external or internal pain, or can be generated from a physical source. For example, you may cut your finger (external) or have a stomachache (internal).

Feelings can be generated outside or inside the body by simply hearing, eating, smelling, tasting, or seeing foods. Such feelings can be considered sensations and are caused by your own personal experiences, reactions, and perceptions of the food. These feelings are established early, during your first contact with a food.

Now let's take a look at the definition of emotions as they relate to food feelings. Emotions are reactions and responses to feelings, life experiences and circumstances, or to someone or something—in this case food. Emotions can be felt in the body and triggered with thoughts originating from our minds, either consciously or unconsciously.

Desires are reactions and can be considered emotions. Cravings can be feelings or emotions, depending on what is experienced during the craving.

Do not worry if you are still a bit confused. You will be given all the information you need in the later chapters on finding food feelings.

Let's look at a few examples of how a food feeling will either motivate you to eat a food or induce you to avoid it.

Examples

A person might see a bag of cookies, hear them mentioned, or just think about cookies, and the food feeling would be triggered unconsciously. Let's say the food feeling for cookies in this example is a sweet sensation in the back of the throat. The feeling would be triggered (activated), and the unconscious feeling would motivate him or her to eat cookies.

The same is also true of foods we dislike. This same person may hear the word cabbage and experience a food feeling for it. The food feeling for cabbage might be a bitter sensation on the tip of the tongue, which would deter the person from buying a head of cabbage and eating it.

Food feelings are triggered and experienced in seconds, and decisions are then made from an unconscious level regarding what to eat or not to eat, as the above examples demonstrate.

You can consciously ignore food feelings temporarily in certain situations, but most of the time you will revert back to them. For example, if you are starving (or very hungry), you will eat something that is available, although it may not be what you normally like. You are able to temporarily ignore the food feeling the food typically evokes.

Furthermore, when you are on a diet, you are constantly trying to overcome food feelings. Diets create continuous internal battles to override food feelings imbedded in your unconscious mind.

Both situations are short-term. Once you are no longer starving or are off the diet, the food feelings programmed in your unconscious mind will once again prevail.

You do not need to be concerned with how and when your food feelings were created and became imbedded in your unconscious mind. It could have happened in childhood or last year; this information is not important or needed for the program to work. All you have to do is become aware of the food feelings you want to change, and then change them for your benefit. That's exactly what this Food Feelings Program will teach you, step by step.

In the next chapter, you will find out how the Food Feelings Program works.

Your stomach shouldn't be a waist basket.

~Author Unknown

Chapter 3

The Four Steps

As explained in the first chapter (page 18), there are key elements needed to make the Food Feelings Program successful. These key elements are acquired through four steps. The following are the steps, and I will discuss each one individually.

The Four Steps

- Identifying the food feeling of the food(s) you like but want to reduce and/or eliminate from your diet.

- Identifying several food feelings of foods you dislike eating.

- Finding the area in the body where your food feelings are located.

- Moving the food feelings to different locations in the body.

The following is an overview of the four steps that make up the Food Feeling Program.

First Step

If you see, smell, think about, or hear the name of a food, a food feeling is experienced and will motivate you to eat or not eat that food. So, for the first step, you must make a list of the food(s) you want to reduce or eliminate from your diet, and then identify their food feelings.

Since food feelings are experienced subliminally in your unconscious mind, you will need to consciously learn the process for becoming aware of, and identifying, these feelings for the foods on your list.

It is important to state again, your food feelings were created in many different ways, but you do not need to know when or why the food feelings were created and imbedded subliminally in your unconscious mind for the program to work.

Since I have mentioned the word subliminal, let's talk about it before we go to the second step. Subliminal is defined as something that functions or exists below the threshold of conscious awareness. That threshold for this program is your unconscious mind, or as it is sometimes called, your subconscious mind.

While your conscious mind can process up to nine thoughts a minute, in that same minute, your unconscious mind processes 2.3 million bits of information. It stores everything in your memory: life experiences, beliefs, and most importantly, all your habits, good and bad.

Besides processing information, your unconscious mind controls many internal body functions without you thinking about it. Your unconscious mind is always working, whether you are awake or asleep.

Second Step
The second step is identical to the first, except you make a small list of several foods you dislike. (Initially, don't start with more than a few). You will use the same process to identify the food feelings on this list.

Third Step
Once you have identified the food feelings for the foods you have on your two lists, the next step is to find the area in the body where they are located.

This might sound strange at first, but everybody has unique locations for food feelings in the body. For some people, ice cream's food feeling location is in the stomach, or the tip of the tongue, or maybe at the back of the throat. A food feeling's location can be anywhere in the body.

There. is no right or wrong location for a food feeling. I have worked with people whose locations are anywhere from inside their elbows to their feet. So the third step is locating where the food feelings are experienced in the body. You will learn a process for accomplishing this.

Fourth Step

The fourth step is to move the food feeling from the location of the food you wish to stop eating to the location of the food you dislike. You will do this with your conscious mind for a few minutes a day for 21 days. During those 21 days, the power of your unconscious mind will eventually imbed the food feeling of the food you want to stop eating into the location of the food you dislike.

After the step is completed, the food feeling for the food you want to stop eating now has some, if not all of the attributes of the food you dislike.

What this means is that in the future, when you hear, smell, see, eat, or think about the food you want to reduce or eliminate from your diet, you will unconsciously experience a similar, if not the same, food feeling for the food you dislike. This will cause you to eat less, or eliminate altogether, the food you want to stop eating, without even thinking about it. You will learn the process for accomplishing this step in the following chapters.

These four steps and the process for performing them comprise the complete Food Feeling Program. In the following chapters, you will learn how to implement the steps and processes that go along with them.

*Eat to live, and
do not live to eat.*

~William Penn, 1693

Chapter 4

The Potential

There are many reasons for starting a Food Feelings Program: health and medical issues, saving money (junk food is not cheap), but the most popular reason is the desire to lose weight. Whatever the reason(s), people like the following aspects of the program that make it unique.

- The program's weight loss potential depends solely on the elimination of certain foods, not on increased physical activity or specialized diet plans. And you can pick the foods you want to work with.

- The program is simple and fun to do.

- The program will lessen caloric intake and thus create weight loss in just five minutes a day for three weeks, without any willpower.

33

- The program can be effective without any other weight loss method. It can also be used in conjunction with a more traditional weight loss program that may employ an exercise regimen and/or diet.

Let's discuss diet plans and calories.

Diet Plans

Many programs and books claim to hold the secrets to weight loss. Some offer high protein and low carbohydrate diets. Others recommend only eating fruits and vegetables. Their success ultimately relies on eating less food and cutting out certain foods in your diet. This means fewer calories and results in weight loss. But you must use willpower to stay on these programs. When you pit willpower against imbedded food feelings, ultimately the food feelings will win, unless you change them.

Fast Weight Loss

Diet plans that include weight loss pills or supplements promoting very fast weight loss—sometimes as much as 4-6 pounds per week—are not typically healthy. (There are exceptions when under medical supervision.)

Studies have shown that an average healthy human body simply will not lose more than about 2-3 pounds of fat per week. But it will shed water, which creates fast weight loss. However, the water weight quickly returns once the program for rapid weight loss is halted. The Food Feelings Program is about losing weight safely, and over a period of time.

Calorie Minimum

The average person's body requires at least 1,200 calories per day to maintain basic body performance. Anything less than that amount may actually cause a person to gain weight. This happens because the body's metabolism is lowered, requiring fewer calories, so the body begins storing fat as quickly as possible. The majority of people who try the Food Feelings Program do not have a problem with the minimum requirement of calories. Junk food always contains high calories, and some people can consume 1,200 or more calories in one snack.

A Pound of Fat

One pound of stored body fat contains 3,500 calories. If a 3,500-calorie deficit is created through diet, one pound of body weight will be lost. A healthy goal is to lose 1-1.5 pounds per week. If you consume 500 calories less each day, it will result in weight loss at a rate of one pound per week, which will put you in the healthy range.

Of course, most of the foods you wish to stop eating, or at least cut back on, are high in calories. By eliminating half the amount of two junk foods you now eat, you will reach that goal for healthy weight loss.

Charts at the end of this chapter will show two scenarios. One scenario is the impact and potential weight loss of eliminating a few junk foods in your diet. The other scenario is the potential weight gain these foods can promote in your diet. When people view these charts, they are amazed that stopping or continuing to eat just a few junk foods can cause such dramatic changes in their weight over a short period of time.

Now here are a few examples of these scenarios.

Potential Weight Gain

Let's use an example of a person who consumes an 18-ounce bag of potato chips a week, every week for a year. At 150 calories per ounce, that amount of chips equals 2,700 calories. Thus, by eating one bag per week for one month, this person consumes 10,800 calories and gains 3 pounds. At three months, 32,400 calories would have been consumed and 9 pounds gained; at six months, 64,000 calories would have been consumed and over 18 pounds gained; at nine months 97,200 calories would have been consumed and 27 pounds gained. In a year's time, an astounding 129,600 calories would have been consumed by eating just one bag of chips a week, which can result in a weight gain of over 37 pounds.

Potential Weight Loss

In terms of potential weight loss, eliminating those 18-ounce bags of potato chips over a one-month period would result in a loss of more than 3 pounds. In a three-month period, about 10 pounds would be lost, and so on. And in a year's time a person could experience a whopping weight loss of over 37 pounds. You can see how the potential for weight loss can add up by eliminating even one junk food from your diet.

Eliminating Half the Calories

Suppose a person reduces the intake of potato chips by only half with the program. Reducing the consumption of half the chips can still make a huge impact on the amount of weight that can potentially be lost over a year. Reducing those 18 ounces of potato chips per week to half in a month's time would be 5,400 fewer calories consumed, in three months 16,200 fewer calories consumed and so on. This will still add up to an impressive weight loss by just cutting the consumption of one food in half.

Let's take it a step further in the following example:

A person has completed the Food Feeling Program for potato chips and has successfully cut back on half the amount of chips being eaten, as in the example explained previously. Now the person decides to apply the program to cookies. Cookies are another high-calorie food that many people consume on a regular basis. This individual calculates that he or she snacks on one bag of Oreo cookies per week. A bag of Oreos has 15 servings (three cookies) with 160 calories per serving, which comes to about 2,400 calories. The person does the program and is able to stop eating

Oreos altogether. After three months, 28,800 fewer calories would be consumed; at six months, 57,600 fewer calories; at nine months, 86,400 fewer calories; and at a year, 115,200 fewer calories would be consumed.

In terms of weight loss, by reducing the intake of half the cookies for three months, your weight loss would be approximately 4 pounds, about 8 pounds at six months, about 12 pounds at nine months, and about 16 pounds after a year. If combined with the weight loss realized by cutting back on the potato chips, you are looking at a significant number of pounds lost in a year by just cutting back on half of these junk foods.

The following lists give samples of junk food and their calories to give you an idea how many calories you are consuming. Make sure you check on the label of the junk food you are eating for the exact amount of calories.

After the lists are a few charts that will open your eyes to the potential weight gain and loss just by eating, or not eating, a few common junk foods.

Cakes	Serving Size	Calories
Coffee cake	2oz slice	260
Crumb cake	2oz slice	220
Cup cake, chocolate	2oz slice	190
Carrot cake w/icing	1 cake (10" dia)	6,100
Cheesecake	1 cake (9" dia)	3,400

Candies	Serving Size	Calories
Gumdrops	1oz	110
Chocolate coated peanuts	1oz	155
Milk chocolate, regular	2 oz	300
Milk chocolate, regular	4 oz	600
Hershey bar	1 (1.5oz)	240
Hershey kisses	9 (1.5oz)	220
M & M's, plain	1 pkt	230
M & M's, peanut	1 pkt	250
Skittles	1 pkt (2.8oz)	250
Snickers bar	1 bar (2.1oz)	280
Caramels	1	31
Caramels, chocolate	1	22
Carob bar	1 3oz	450
Jelly beans	1oz	105

Chips	Serving Size	Calories
Corn chips, plain	7oz	1,067
Corn chips, barbecue	7oz	1,036
Corn puffs, cheese chips	8oz	1,256
Potato chips	8oz	1,210
Potato chips, light	6oz	801
Potato chips, cream & onion	7oz	1,051
Tortilla chips	7.5oz	1,067
Nacho chips	8oz	1,130
Potato sticks	1oz	148

Cookies	No of Cookies	Calories
Animal crackers	1	11
Chocolate chip cookies	1	48
Chocolate wafer cookies	1	26

Cookies (continued)	No of Cookies	Calories
Ginger snap cookies	1	29
Graham chocolate cookies	1	68
Fortune cookies	1	30
Oatmeal raisin cookies	1	81
Shortbread cookies	1	40
Biscotti cookies	1	127
Peanut butter sandwich cookies	1	67
Vanilla sandwich cookies	1	48

Danish Pastries	Serving Size	Calories
Almond danish	2.5oz	280
Apple danish	2.5oz	265
Cheese danish	2.5oz	265
Cinnamon danish	2.5oz	260
Coffee danish	2.5oz	220
Plain danish	2.5oz	220

Donuts	Serving Size	Calories
Plain donuts	1 (1.5oz)	165
Cake-type unsugared donuts	1 (1.6oz)	198
Chocolate coated donuts	1 (1.5oz)	204
Chocolate sugared donuts	1 (1.5oz)	175
Creme-filled donuts	1 (3oz)	307
Frosted donuts	1 (1.5oz)	204
Honey-bun donuts	1 (2.1oz)	242
Jelly donuts	1 (3oz)	289
Old-fashioned donuts	1 (1.6oz)	198
Sugared donuts	1 (1.6oz)	192

French Fries	Serving Size	Calories
French fries	Large	540
French fries	Super	610
French fries	Medium	390
French fries	Small	257

Ice Cream	Serving Size	Calories
Vanilla ice cream	1/2 cup	132

Vanilla rich ice cream	1/2 cup	178
Chocolate ice cream	1/2 cup	143
Butter pecan ice cream	1/2 cup	310
Strawberry ice cream	1/2 cup	127
Chocolate chip ice cream	1/2 cup	270
Coffee ice cream	1/2 cup	290
Vanilla fudge ice cream	1/2 cup	290
Ice cream, soft-serve, regular	1/2 cup	140

Onion Rings	Serving Size	Calories
Onion rings	Small	180
Onion rings	Medium	320
Onion rings	Large	480

Pretzels	Serving Size	Calories
Pretzels generic	1oz	108
Soft pretzels	2.25oz	170
Pretzel sticks	1oz	115

Quesadillas	Serving Size	Calories
Quesadilla (generic)	1 x 6"	430

Shake	Serving Size	Calories
Chocolate shake (generic)	10oz	360
Strawberry shake (generic)	10oz	319
Vanilla shake (generic)	10oz	314

Sodas	Serving Size	Calories
Coca-Cola	12 fl oz	150
Coca-Cola	16 fl oz	200
Coca-Cola	20 fl oz	250
Lemon lime	12 fl oz	220
Orange	12 fl oz	180
Root beer	12 fl oz	165

Sugar	Serving Size	Calories
Table Sugar	1 teaspoon (6g)	25Table
Sugar	1 cup	770

FRENCH FRIES

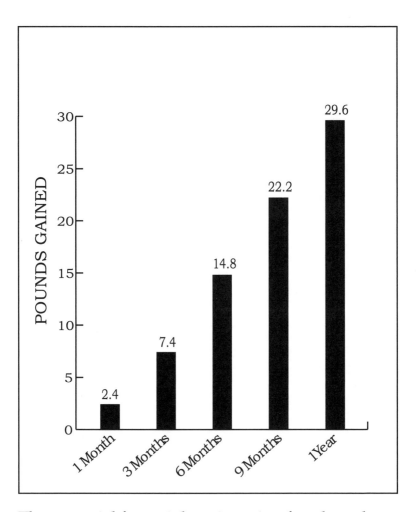

The potential for weight gain eating four large bags of fries a week. Each bag of fries has 540 calories.

FRENCH FRIES

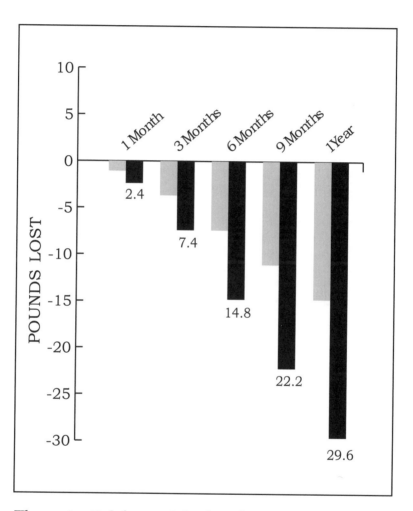

The potential for weight loss by eating half (gray bar) or eliminating completely (black bar) four large bags of fries a week from your diet. Each bag of fries has 540 calories.

FROSTED DONUT

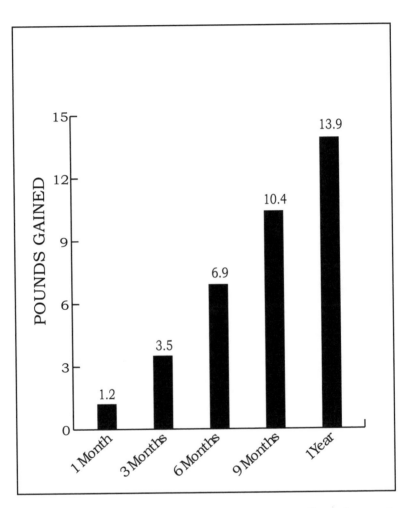

The potential for weight gain eating five frosted donuts a week. Each donut is 1.5 oz. and has 204 calories.

FROSTED DONUT

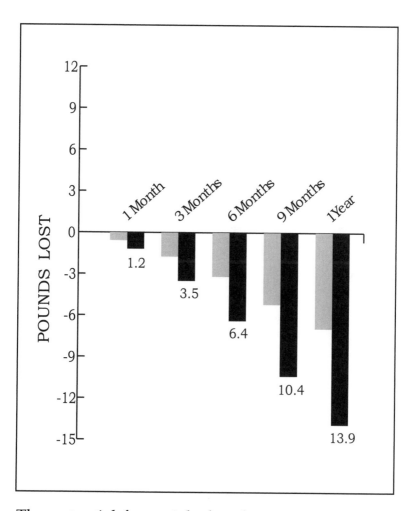

The potential for weight loss by eating half (gray bar) or eliminating completely (black bar) five frosted donuts a week from your diet. Each donut is 1.5 oz. and has 204 calories.

CHOCOLATE BAR

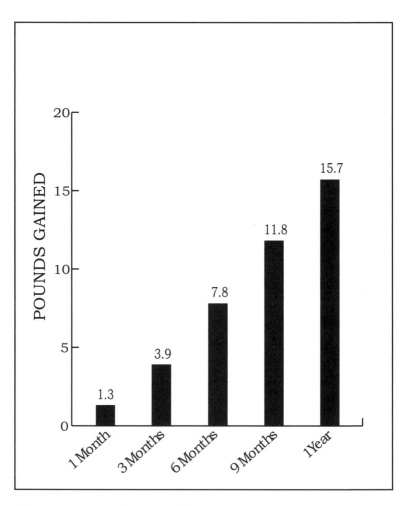

The potential for weight gain eating five chocolate bars a week. Each donut is 1.5 oz. and has 230 calories.

CHOCOLATE BAR

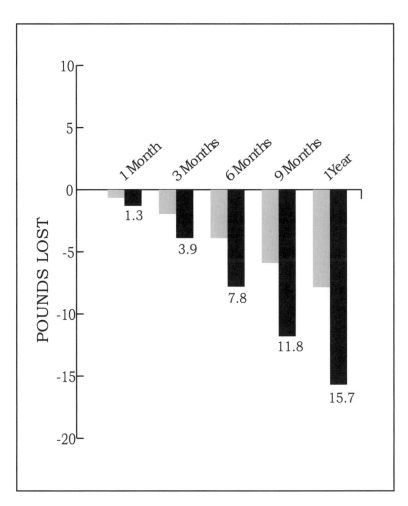

The potential for weight loss by eating half (gray bar) or eliminating completely (black bar) five chocolate bars a week from your diet. Each donut is 1.5 oz. and has 230 calories.

Rich, fatty foods
are like destiny:
they too, shape our ends.

~Author Unknown

Chapter 5

Preparation

Before you learn how to prepare for the Food Feelings Program, I will discuss the varying degrees of success you can have with it. The program is more of an art than a science. Since everybody is different, the results will vary with each food and each individual when it comes to food feelings. You may cut back on half of the junk food in your diet or eliminate it all together, or you may fall somewhere in between.

As the charts in the last chapter show, even a 50 percent reduction of one to three regularly consumed high-calorie foods can generate significant weight loss over the upcoming months and years of your life.

The Food Feelings Program can help you

achieve your weight loss goal.

Preparing for the Program

To begin the program, there are several things you need to learn and do. Once you accomplish these, you will only need five minutes a day for 21 days to complete the program. You will be able to do the program anywhere: at the office, the gym, even in the bathroom.

Visual or Non-Visual

First of all, it is important to establish if you are visual or non-visual. This comes into play while you are implementing the program. To find out which type you are, take the following easy test:

Close your eyes and relax for a few moments. Imagine being at your favorite place. This can be outdoors, a friend's house, the gym, your parents' house, etc. You can imagine being anywhere you like. Now, while you are imagining this, can you see your surroundings? If so describe what you see to yourself. If you cannot see what you are imagining, still describe the place to yourself. You will find that although you cannot visualize the location, you can still describe the place. If you were able to see your favorite place, then you are visual. If you could not see it, but were able to describe it, you are non-visual.

Food Lists

Next, get a pen or pencil and a pad of paper, and make a list like the example that is provided on the following page (Chart 9). The list will offer examples and will be updated and shown throughout the book. You will use the same type of list but with your choices and results.

Now list three foods that you would like to stop or reduce in your diet and prioritize them, beginning with the item you would most like to eliminate. For example, let's suppose you have listed potato chips, ice cream, and chocolate cake. The food you most want eliminated is potato chips, the second ice cream, and the third chocolate cake. Always work with the first junk food you want eliminated or reduced before moving down the list. If you have more than three foods you want to reduce or stop eating, work on them only after the first three are done. If you only have one or two foods to work with, just list those.

Next, estimate how much of these foods you eat in a month and write it down. This does not have to be exact, just your best honest guess. Follow the list in the book as an example. The list will help you track your progress and the success with the food(s) you are using in this program.

Now make a list of one or two foods that you dislike eating. I have yet to find a person who did not have at least one food he or she disliked. But if you are a person who likes every type of food, then make a list of one or two foods you like the least. For example, you might list green beans because you do not eat them often.

Let's say the two foods you listed were green

CHART 9

Foods You Want To Stop Eating	30 Days	Food Feeling	Location
1. Potato chips	10 bags		
2. Ice cream	30 scoops		
3. Chocolate cake	14 slices		

Foods You Dislike	30 Days	Food Feeling	Location
1. Green beans	none		
2. Cabbage	2 servings		

beans and cabbage. Next, you would rank the foods according to which you like the least, starting with number one. In this scenario, green beans, being the least liked, would be number one followed by cabbage.

You now have the first list of foods that you will use in your Food Feelings Program.

Relaxation Technique

Now you must learn a quick relaxation technique that you will use each time you work with the Food Feelings Program. It is simple, easy to learn, and only takes about two minutes from start to finish.

This technique will not relax you into a deep meditation or put you to sleep. It was designed to quickly ease the body, and then the mind, into a state of light relaxation. When you are in this light state of relaxation, it is easier for you to work with your unconscious mind and food feelings.

Once you become accustomed to performing the relaxation technique, you will find yourself slipping into this relaxed state more quickly each time you do it. And you will be able to do it anywhere at anytime. Some people like the relaxation technique so well, they use it before, during, or after any stressful situation they might encounter.

Relaxation Instructions

Find a place where you will not be disturbed for a few minutes and get into a comfortable position.

1. Close your eyes and take five easy deep breaths, focusing on really filling up the lungs. On each exhale, say the word "relax" silently. When you are done with the five breaths, just resume your normal breathing and stop saying the word relax.

2. Next, with your eyes still closed, simultaneously tense or tighten your entire upper body the best you can: arms, chest, neck, hands, etc. Tightening your upper body might seem awkward at first for some people, but with practice you will soon become an expert at it. Keep your upper body tense for about 30 seconds, then release the tension and let your upper body relax and go limp for 30 seconds. While you are doing this, just continue to breathe at your own pace.

3. With your eyes still closed, simultaneously tense or tighten your entire lower body the best you can: hips, legs, calves, feet, etc. Tense them for 30 seconds, then release the tension and relax, allowing the lower body to go limp for 30 seconds. After that, take three more deep breaths, and you are finished with the technique.

You have now learned the relaxation technique that will be used for the first two minutes of your five-minute Food Feelings Program.

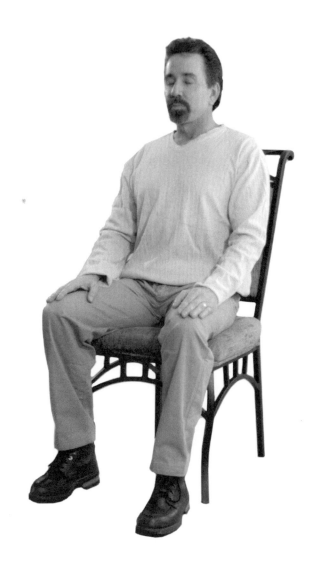

1. Close your eyes and take five nice, easy, deep breaths, focusing on really filling up the lungs. On each exhale, say the word "relax" silently.

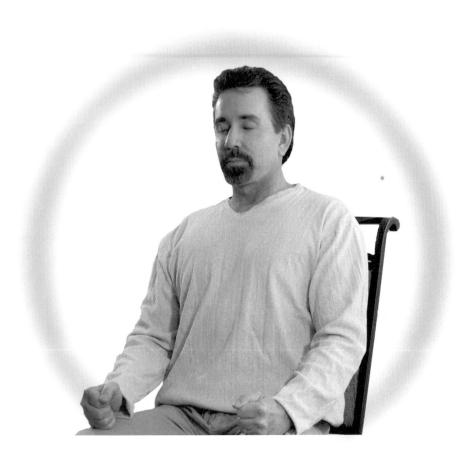

2. Simultaneously tense or tighten your entire upper body the best you can: arms, chest, neck hands, etc.

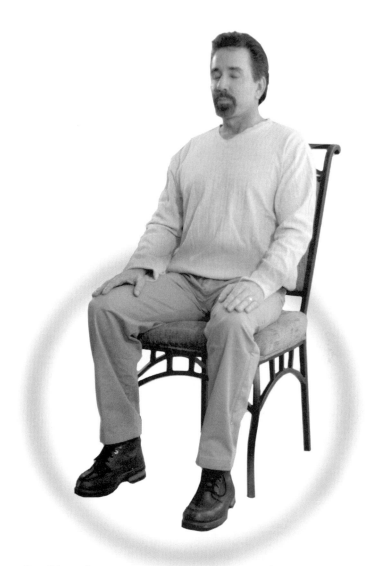

3. Simultaneously tense or tighten your entire lower body the best you can: hips, legs, calves, feet, etc.

To lengthen your life,
shorten your meals.

~Unknown Author

Chapter 6

Identifying Food Feelings

To identify and locate your food feelings, find a quiet room where you will not be disturbed for a while.

As I mentioned before, you can only do the 21-day program for one food at a time, so take a look at your list of foods you want to stop eating and pick the one at the top. Then take a look at the list of the foods you dislike and choose the one at the top of that list.

Now place the two foods you selected with you in the room. For example, if you are going to stop eating potato chips, have a few chips available, and if the food you dislike is green beans, have a few green beans available.

Because identifying and finding your food feelings may seem awkward or strange at first, it might take you a bit longer the first few times to identify food feelings.

After you identify the feelings a few times and become accustomed to the process, it will become easy and only take a few minutes to do.

Identifying Food Feelings

Once you are in a quiet room, set the food you want to stop eating in front of you. This can be on a table, stand, etc. You can hold the food in your hand, but with some foods that will be difficult. For obvious reasons, you should put such foods as ice cream or cake in a dish.

Look at the food for a few seconds, then close your eyes and think about what you are feeling or experiencing when you see the food. Do not strain or worry about doing this right. Remember, it can take longer the first few times.

If, after a minute or so, you cannot discover the feeling, open your eyes and look at the food for a few seconds, then close your eyes and do it again. Do this until you become aware of a feeling associated with the food and are able to identify it. It should only take you a few tries to become aware of the feeling, even if you are new to the process. Once you are experienced at identifying a food feeling, you will be able to close your eyes and do it in 10–15 seconds.

The first feeling you experience is the one you are looking for. It is this initial feeling about the food that will be the most valid. Once you identify this first feeling, stop. Do not dwell on it, analyze it, or second-guess it. That is your food feeling for this food. Write it down on your list next to the junk food. Remember, a food feeling can be different for every person, as described in chapter two.

The following chart lists a few examples of common food feelings for junk foods that are liked. You might find feelings for the foods you have chosen on the chart. Or your food feelings may not be listed; if that is the case, write down the ones you identify. Please note, as some examples show, a food feeling can be a combination of feelings.

Common Food Feelings for Foods You Like

Happiness	Satisfaction	Pleasure
Sweetness	Comfort	Enjoyment
Excitement	Warmness	Fulfillment
Gratification	Contentment	Blissfulness
Warm-Tingly	Velvety-Sweet	Silky-Soft
Cozy-Warm	Full-Content	Happy-Pleasing

The next step is to do the same process for the food you dislike. You will put the food in front of you, close your eyes and identify its food feeling.

Once you discover the feeling write it down.

The following chart lists a few examples of common food feelings for foods that are disliked. You might find yours there, or you might not. Either way, write down the ones you identify.

Again, please note, as some examples show, a food feeling can be a combination of feelings.

Common Food Feelings for Foods You Dislike

Slimy	Distasteful	Bitterness
Salty	Coldness	Blandness
Spicy	Nausea	Tart
Vinegary	Greasy-Tasteless	Curdled-Pungent
Spoiled-Vinegary	Nasty-Soggy	Irritating-Squishy
Oily-Pungent	Soggy-Plain	Repulsive-Foul

Examples

Let's look at an example of this process. You want to stop eating potato chips, so that's what you place in front of you.

Look at the chips (photo #4) then close your eyes. With eyes closed, you become aware of and identify a happy feeling (photo #5) associated with the chips. Happiness is your food feeling for the potato chips; jot that down (chart #10) next to potato chips on your list.

The same process (photo #7 and #8) for green beans (the food you dislike) is applied, and a food feeling of bitterness is identified. Write this down on the list (chart #11).

You have two food feelings for the foods you are working with; now it's on to the next step and process.

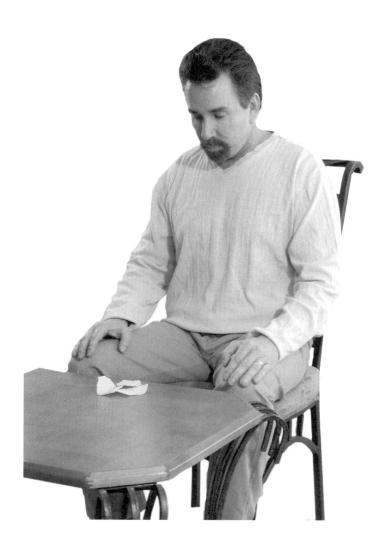

Photo #4

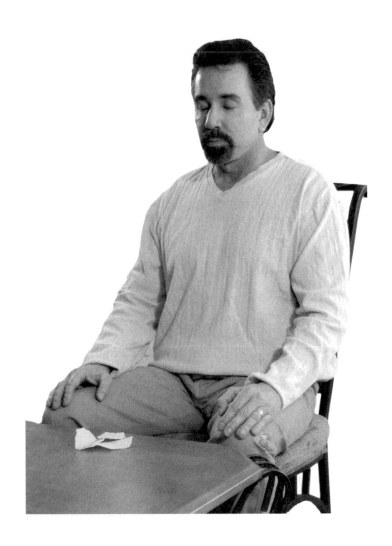

Photo #5

CHART 10

Foods You Want To Stop Eating	30 Days	Food Feeling	Location
1. Potato chips	10 bags	happiness	
2. Ice cream	30 scoops		
3. Chocolate cake	14 slices		

Foods You Dislike	Food Feeling	Location
1. Green beans	none	
2. Cabbage	2 servings	

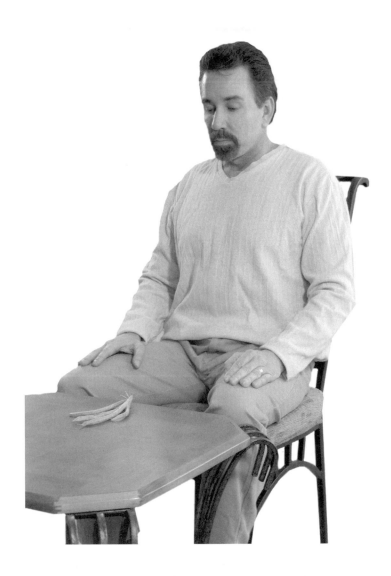

Photo #7

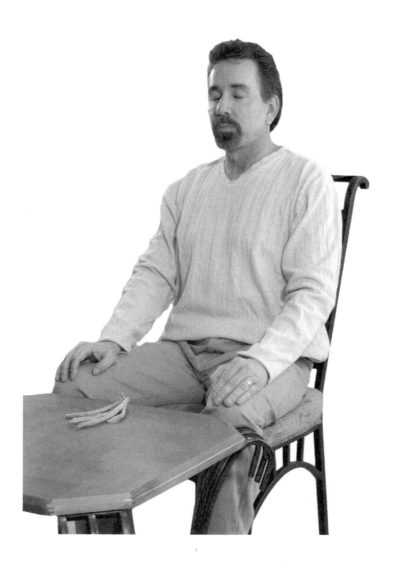

Photo #8

CHART 11

Foods You Want To Stop Eating	30 Days	Food Feeling	Location
1. Potato chips	10 bags	happiness	
2. Ice cream	30 scoops		
3. Chocolate cake	14 slices		

Foods You Dislike	Food Feeling	Location	
1. Green beans	none	bitterness	
2. Cabbage	2 servings		

*We rarely repent of
having eaten too little.*

~Thomas Jefferson

A bagel is a doughnut

with the sin removed.

~George Rosenbaum

Chapter 7

Locating Food Feelings

The next process is fun, although it might seem different at first. But once you do it a few times, it will become easy.

Now that you know the two food feelings (happiness and bitterness) for the foods you are working with, you need to find where you store these feelings in your body. When I first tell people this, I always receive puzzled looks. But after they locate their food feelings a few times in their bodies, they laugh and are amazed at how easy it is and how they were never aware of them before.

Next, look at the potato chips again, close your eyes and become aware of the food feeling for them. In this example it is a feeling of happiness.

Now that you are experiencing the feeling, where is the feeling located in your body? In other words, where do you feel, know, or sense its location? After about 30 seconds, you discover that the happiness feeling (photo #9) is located in the middle of your stomach.

What I am asking you to do might seem different and new. I promise that after the first few times of trying this process, it will not be a problem for the majority of people to discover the location of food feelings in their bodies. With a bit more practice, the rest of you will eventually succeed, and then be able to do it quickly. Just stay relaxed and take your time the first few times you try this process.

Please do not be surprised by the location of these feelings. People have had food feelings located in elbows and even in their feet; there is never a right or wrong location for a food feeling.

Just like the previous process, it might take a few tries before you are successful. After you become experienced with the process, it should only take about 15-30 seconds to find a food feeling's location.

If you are initially confused about this process, or cannot locate the area for the food feeling after a few minutes and several tries, here's what you do:

Take a deep breath, open your eyes briefly, and

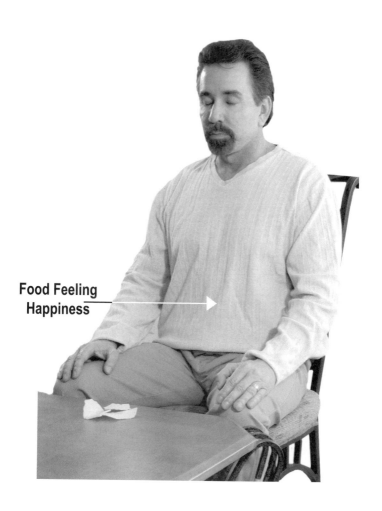

**Food Feeling
Happiness**

Photo #9

look at the food you are trying to reduce or eliminate from your diet. Then close your eyes and guess or just imagine where the food feeling is located in your body. Use whatever location first comes to mind.

For example, if you are stuck and cannot locate the area, perform the above process. Write down the first location that comes to mind (for example, in the middle of your throat).

Both methods will work in finding the location of food feelings, and these locations will be effective in your Food Feelings Program. With practice, you will be able to use the first method of closing your eyes and finding the location directly.

Location of Foods You Dislike

You will use the same process for finding food feeling locations for the foods you dislike. Look at the green beans and close your eyes, becoming aware of the food feeling for them. In this case it is a bitterness feeling.

Now that you are experiencing the feeling, where is the feeling located in your body? Where do you feel, know, or sense its location? After about 30 seconds, you discover that the bitterness food feeling (photo #10) is located in the back of your tongue.

Food feelings for foods you dislike generally are located more quickly.

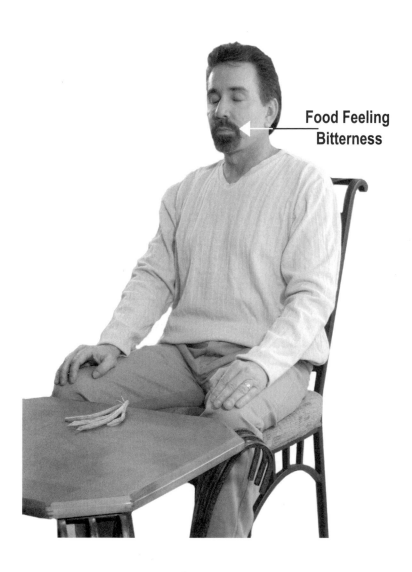

Photo #10

Once you have a location (chart #12) for a food feeling, open your eyes and write it on your list.

Similar Locations

On a few occasions, the location of food feelings for foods you like and dislike might seem to be in the same location, but they are not.

If that happens, you need to pinpoint the specific location in that same area. For example, if the food feelings for both foods are located in the stomach, you need to identify exactly what area of the stomach: the bottom part, middle, top part, or lower right area, etc.

To do this, you need to close your eyes again and pinpoint the exact area in the stomach where the feeling of the food you like is located. Then do the same for the food you dislike.

Let's take an example all the way through to show this process.

The food feelings for both foods you are working with are found in the stomach. First, close your eyes to determine the specific area for the food feeling you like. You discover it is actually in the top left part (photo #11) of the stomach. Write it down on your list. Next, close your eyes again and do the same for the food you dislike. You find this exact location (photo #12) is at the bottom left part of your stomach. Write it down.

In the next chapter, you'll find the final step and process for the Food Feelings Program.

CHART 12

Foods You Want To Stop Eating	30 Days	Food Feeling	Location
1. Potato chips	10 bags	happiness	middle of stomach
2. Ice cream	30 scoops		
3. Chocolate cake	14 slices		

Foods You Dislike	Food Feeling	Location	
1. Green beans	none	bitterness	back of tongue
2. Cabbage	2 servings		

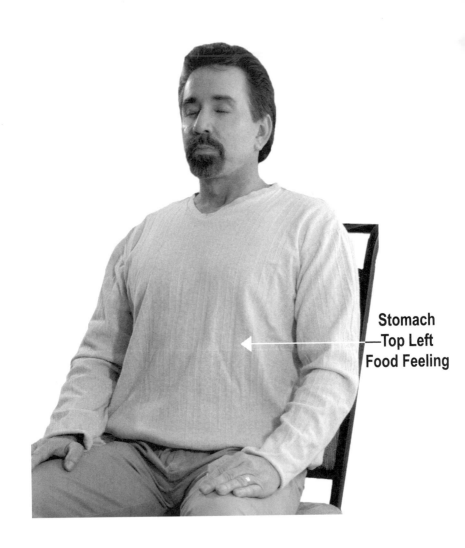

Stomach
—Top Left
Food Feeling

Photo #11

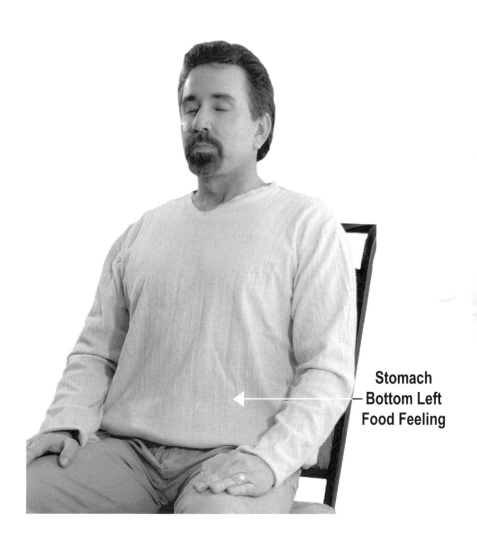

**Stomach
— Bottom Left
Food Feeling**

Photo #12

Tell me what you eat,

I'll tell you who you are.

~Anthelme Brillat-Savarin

Chapter 8

The Program

Now the fun part of the program starts. You have discovered if you are visual or non-visual, learned a quick relaxation technique, and have identified two food feelings: one for a food you want to cut back on or stop eating, the other for a food you dislike eating or eat very little of. You have also located these two food feelings in your body. Now you are all set for the last step of the program.

Guidelines

The following are guidelines for the last process of the Food Feeling Program:

- Do this part of the program for 21 consecutive days; if you miss a day, start over. This is very important. It takes 21 days for the food feeling to become imbedded in its new location in your unconscious mind.

- You can implement the program anywhere and at anytime during the day, as long as you will not be disturbed for five minutes. However, before you take your program "on the road," do it a few times in the same area and at the same time each day until you are comfortable with the process.

- For the first few days, set aside enough time for the program so you do not feel rushed. You might need some additional time at first. Initially, many people find that it is easier to do the program first thing in the morning or at night before going to bed. With practice, you will be able to do it whenever and wherever there is an opportunity.

- When performing this first step, find a room with a comfortable place to sit or lie down (although sitting up, if possible, is recommended).

- Before you start the 21-day program, review from your list the two food feelings you will be working with and their locations in your body. Now you are ready to begin.

The 1st Day

From your preparation, you are aware of the food feelings and their locations within your body.

Close your eyes and start the two-minute relaxation technique. Make sure that you take very deep breaths, but don't strain yourself.

With your eyes still closed—they stay closed throughout the entire five-minute process—focus on the food feeling of the food you want to stop eating and its location.

We will use our example of potato chips:

The food feeling for potato chips is a happiness feeling located in the middle of your stomach. You focus on the (photo #13) food feeling (happiness) at the location (middle of the stomach) for about a minute. When I say focus, it means to identify the food feeling and its location. You do not have to look at the food to accomplish this. Since you are now aware of its feeling and location, you just have to think about the food to bring up this information.

After about a minute of doing this, clear your mind, and with your eyes still closed, quickly shift your focus to the food feeling of the food you dislike (photo #14) and its location in your body. We will use the example of green beans:

The food feeling for green beans is bitterness and it is located at the back of your tongue. Think about the food and then focus on its food feeling (bitterness) in the appropriate location (back of the tongue) for about a minute.

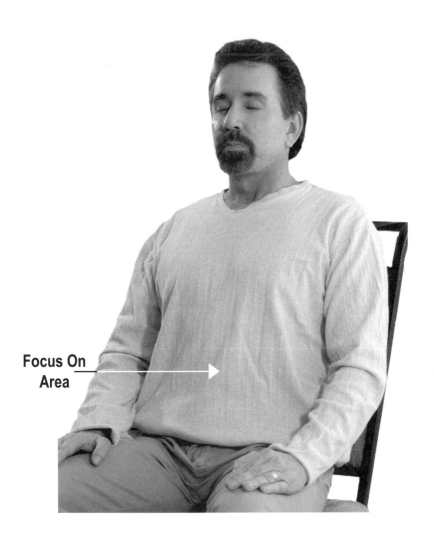

Focus On
Area

Photo #13

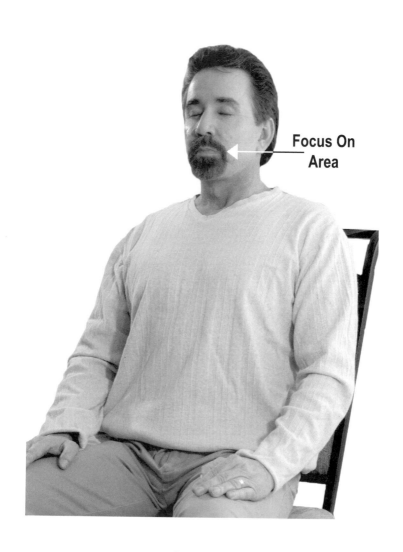

Focus On
Area

Photo #14

After a minute, proceed to the next step, which is very important. The way you will perform it depends on if you are visual or non-visual.

Visual Method

Let's start with the visual method. You are still focused on the food feeling of the food you dislike and its location in your body. Now, visualize a circle around the area (photo #15) of this food feeling, enclosing it entirely. If you are visual, you will be able to see the circle. The circle can be any color, but its size has to be big enough to encircle the entire food feeling at the location.

People who are visual usually do this rapidly, but it may take a little bit longer the first few times. If you are visual, you also have the option of using the same techniques as a non-visual person. Use whichever method works best for you.

Non-Visual Method

If you are non-visual, you still must place the circle around the food feeling, but of course you cannot visualize (see) it. You draw the circle by knowing it's there and by using your thoughts, feelings, words and/or imagination. For example, I am non-visual, so when I do the process I just know the circle is there with my thoughts. Non-visual people will draw the circle in a way that best suits them.

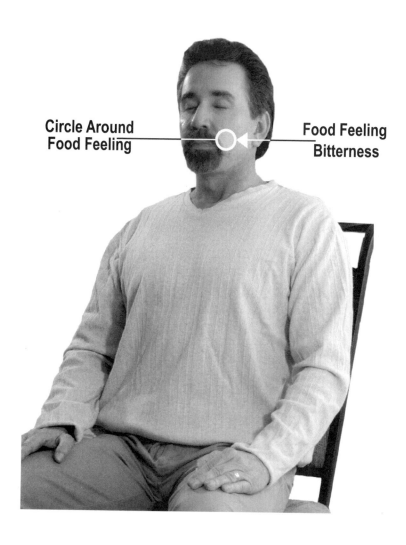

Photo #15

1st Day, Moving the Circle

You have now mentally drawn a circle around the food feeling of the food you dislike. Move this circle to the exact location of the food feeling for the junk food you are now working with.

In our example, you would move the circle around the food feeling at the back of your tongue (green beans) to the area in the middle (photo #16) of your stomach where your food feeling for potato chips is located. It does not matter if the circle is larger than the target area it is moved to. It can and will overlap the area at times, and that is OK.

If you are visual, you can move the circle any way you like. You can move it by seeing it, feeling it, thinking it, or knowing that you moved it. Move the circle the way that works best for you. Most visual people actually see the circle move to the new area, while some people just imagine the circle instantly appearing in the new area. No matter which method you use, moving the circle should only take 15 to 30 seconds at the most, although the first few times might take longer.

If you are non-visual, do the same process, except when you move the circle to the new location, do it with your thoughts, feelings, words, and/or imagination, the same way you drew the circle. Remember, it does not matter if the circle is bigger than the area it is moved to, just place it there.

K!

s simply means is that when you
smell, or taste the junk food you
ng, you will experience the food
od you dislike. In the example
od feeling (happiness) for potato
by the food feeling (bitterness) of
will cause you to automatically
r potato chips. And you will cut
ng them altogether.

re you will not be disturbed for

yes and do the two-minute
que.

l closed, focus on the circle
od feeling you previously moved.
on this food feeling in its new
xt three minutes. Of course, the
t will depend on if you are visual

mple of green beans:

0 days, after you do the two-
technique, focus intensely on
18) now in your stomach with
bitterness) for green beans. Do
nutes. That's all there is to it.
the next 20 days, after the two-
n technique, think of green
on the bitterness food feeling in
stomach for three minutes.

92

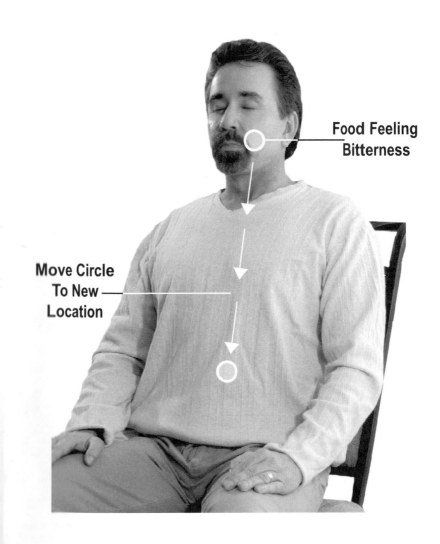

Food Feeling
Bitterness

Move Circle
To New
Location

Photo #16

89

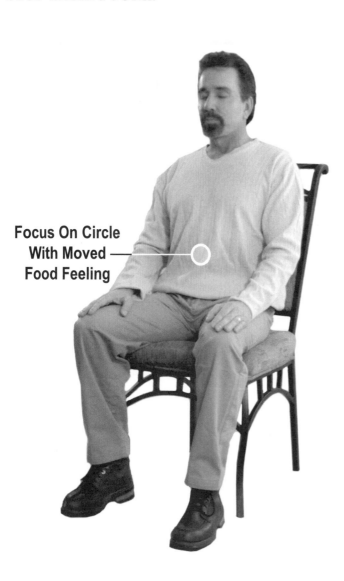

**Focus On Circle
With Moved ——
Food Feeling**

Photo #17

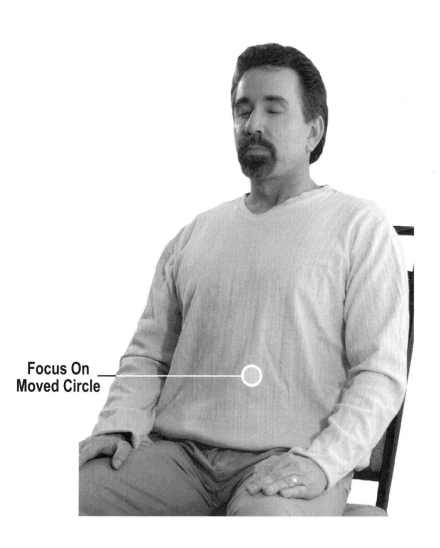

Focus On
Moved Circle

Photo #18

After three minutes of focusing, take a deep breath, open your eyes and you are done. Do this five-minute process once a day for the next 20 days. You only need to do the process once a day, but if you like, you can do it a few more times during the day.

Step-by-Step Review
1st day

1. Go over the food feelings and their locations of the two foods you will be working with from your list. One for the food you want to stop eating and one for the food you dislike.

2. Find a room or an area with no distractions. Make sure there is a comfortable place to sit or lie down. You can lie down, but sitting up, is highly recommended.

3. Now close your eyes and start the two-minute relaxation technique. Make sure that when you take the breaths, they are as deep as possible without straining yourself.

4. Next, with your eyes still closed—they stay closed throughout the entire five-minute process—focus on the food feeling of the food you want to stop eating and its location. We will use our example of potato chips: the food feeling of potato chips is happiness and is located in the middle of your stomach. So you would focus on this food feeling (happiness) in the middle of your stomach.

5. After about a minute, clear your mind and quickly shift your focus to the food feeling of the food you dislike and its location in your body. We will use the example of green beans. The food feeling for green beans (bitterness) is located in the back of your tongue.

6. You are still focused on the food feeling for the food you dislike and its location in your body. Now, mentally draw a circle around the area of this food feeling, enclosing it entirely. Do this whichever way works best for you, visually or non-visually. The circle can be any color, but its size has to be big enough to encircle the entire food feeling.

7. You now have mentally drawn a circle around the food feeling of the food you dislike. Next, move this circle, (visually or non-visually) with the enclosed food feeling to the food feeling location of the junk food.

8. It should only take a few minutes to do this. Once the circle with the food feeling is completely moved to the new area (completely is the key word), continue to focus on the circle and the food feeling at this new area for another 30 seconds. Then take a few deep breaths and open your eyes. You are done for the first day.

Next 20 Days:
1. Find an area where you will not be disturbed for five minutes while doing the process.

2. Close your eyes and do the two-minute relaxation technique.

3. With eyes still closed, focus on the circle with the food feeling you have previously moved to the new location in your body. Focus intensely on this food feeling in its new area for the next three minutes.

4. After three minutes, take a deep breath, open your eyes, and you are done. Do this five-minute process once a day for the next 20 days.

If we're not willing to settle for

junk living, we certainly

shouldn't settle for junk food.

~Sally Edwards

If you want to make

an apple pie from scratch,

you must first

create the universe.

~Carl Sagan

Chapter 9

After The Program

It takes about 30 days after completing the 21-day Food Feelings Program to determine what your final results will be. During those days, keep a record of your contact with the chosen junk food. At the end of the 30 days, compare the record with the list you made before the program.

At this time you might have completely stopped eating the junk food and the program is no longer necessary for this food, except when a Reinforcement Technique is needed.

Or you might eat less of the junk food you previously ate, and you are satisfied with the results. Again the program is no longer necessary for this food, except when a Reinforcement Technique is needed.

If you now eat less of the junk food you previously ate, and you would like to improve on that, just repeat the program again. The results will improve the second time around. After the second program, if improvement is still desired, just do the Reinforcement Technique for this food. Also keep in mind that the benefits of the Food Feelings Program will usually increase with time and you can always do the Reinforcement Technique when needed.

Reinforcement Technique

On occasion, a person might feel the desire to start eating the food that she or he eliminated or reduced from his or her diet. It's the same desire a person experiences when he or she has stopped smoking for years and all of a sudden has a craving to smoke. This desire can be triggered by smelling smoke, seeing or thinking about a cigarette, or simply being in a situation where one usually smokes. The same circumstances can occur with the foods you have worked with in this program.

Anytime you experience a desire, just do the same five-minute process you performed during the 21-day program for that food, three days in a row. You can do this when you first feel the desire for the food or right before you eat it. If you find yourself eating the food, try to do the process while you are eating. This usually will limit the amount of food you consume because it is difficult to eat and do the program at the same time. If for any reason you are unable to accomplish this task, at least implement the technique as soon as possible and continue for the next three days. Using this Reinforcement Technique will put you back on track. You can use this technique as many times as needed.

Additional Programs

After you have completed a Food Feelings Program for one junk food, begin another. You can work on eliminating as many junk foods as you like from your diet, but only do one Food Feelings Program at a time. Always allow a few days before starting a new program.

The last chapter presents the complete program and process in sequence with step-by-step photos.

It's difficult to think
anything but pleasant thoughts
while eating a

homegrown tomato.

~Lewis Grizzard

Chapter 10
_____

Step by Step

The photos in this chapter will assist you in learning and implementing the Food Feelings Program. The photos are in sequence and contain a brief text overview of the complete program and process. The brief text overview is just that; if you need more detailed descriptions of a step, please refer back to the chapter where it was first introduced.

Throughout this chapter the previous examples of potato chips and green beans are used.

Relaxation Technique

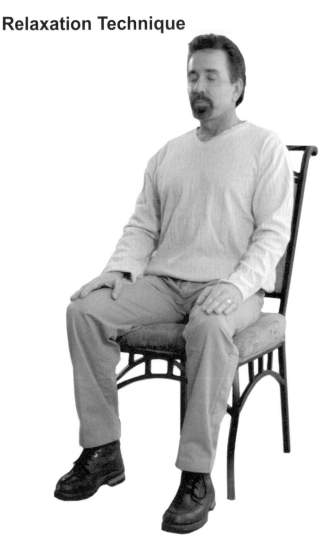

1. Close your eyes and take five nice, deep breaths, focusing on really filling up the lungs. On each exhale, say the word "relax" silently. When you are done with the five breaths, just resume your normal breathing and stop saying the word "relax."

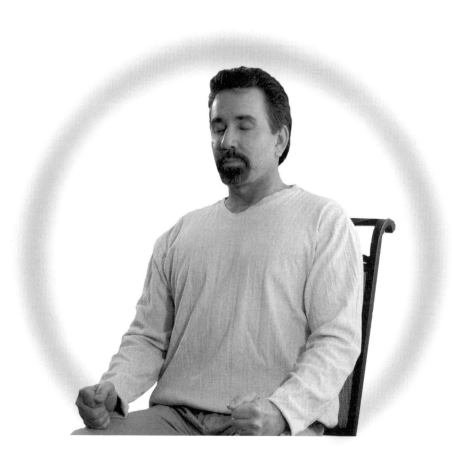

2. Next, with your eyes still closed, simultaneously tense or tighten your entire upper body the best you can: arms, chest, neck, hands, etc. Keep your upper body tense for 30 seconds, then release the tension and let your upper body go limp for 30 seconds.

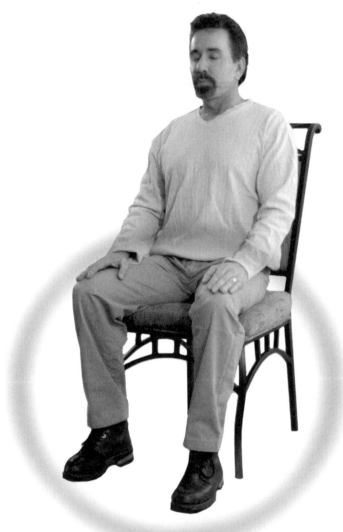

3. Now do the same for your lower body: legs, feet, hips, etc. Tense them for 30 seconds, then release the tension and relax, allowing the lower body to go limp for 30 seconds. After that, take three more deep breaths, and you are finished.

Identifying Food Feelings

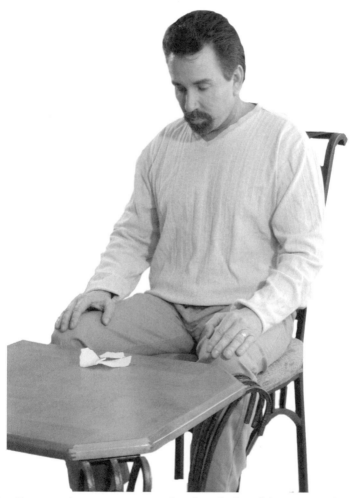

1. In a quiet room, set the junk food (potato chips) you want to stop eating in front of you. Look at the junk food for a few seconds.

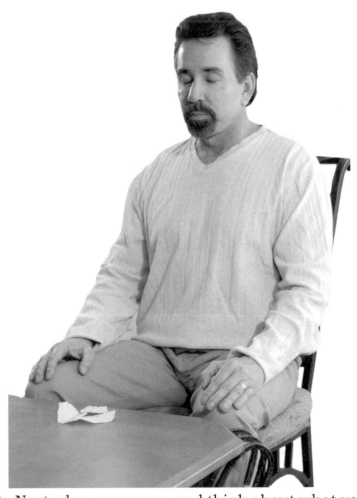

2. Next, close your eyes and think about what you are feeling or experiencing when you see the chips. The first feeling you experience is the one you are looking for. Once you identify the food feeling stop and write it down.

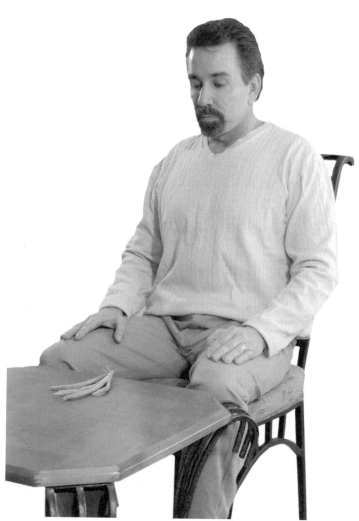

3. Next, set the food you dislike eating (green beans) in front of you. Look at the food for a few seconds.

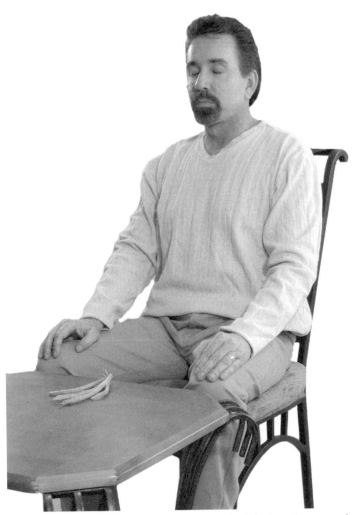

4.   Then close your eyes and think about what you are feeling or experiencing when you see the green beans. Use the first feeling you experience. Once you identify the food feeling stop and write it down.

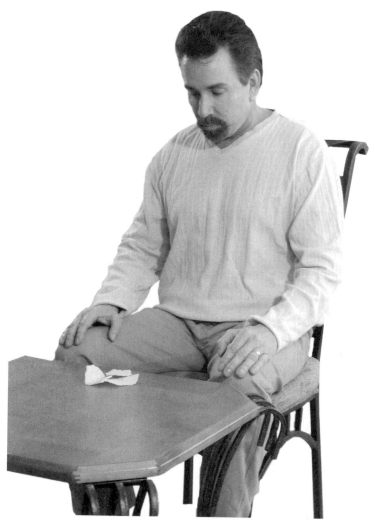

5. Look at the food you want to stop eating (potato chips) again. Close your eyes and identify and experience the food feeling.

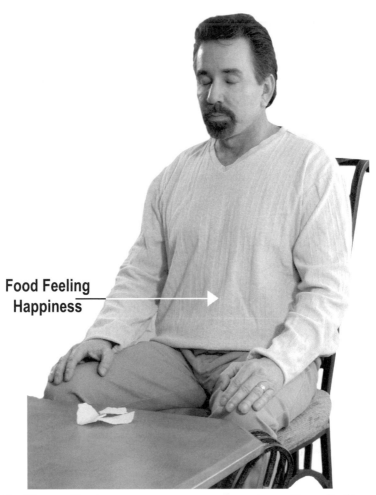

Food Feeling
Happiness

6. Now that you are experiencing the feeling, where is the feeling located (our example, happiness, middle of the stomach) in your body? Where do you feel, know, or sense its location? Write it down.

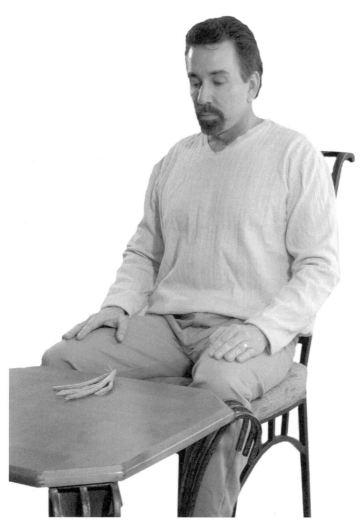

7. Next, look at the food you dislike again, closing your eyes and becoming aware of the food feeling for it.

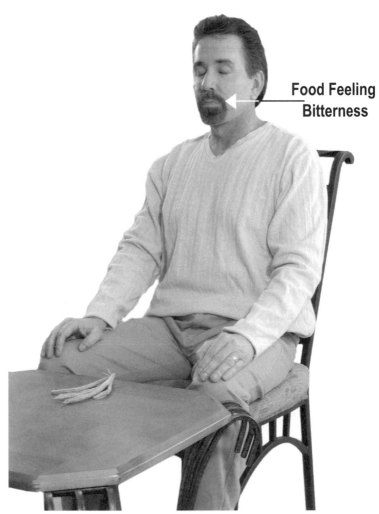

**Food Feeling
Bitterness**

8. Now that you are experiencing the feeling, where is the feeling located (our example, bitterness, back of the tongue) in your body? Where do you feel, know, or sense its location? Write it down.

Food Feelings Program
1st Day

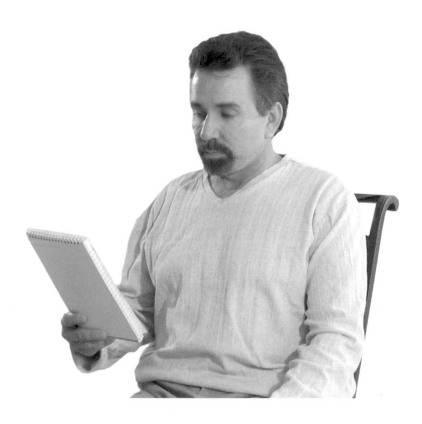

1. Go over the food feelings and their locations of the two foods you will be working with from your list. One for the food you want to stop eating and one for the food you dislike.

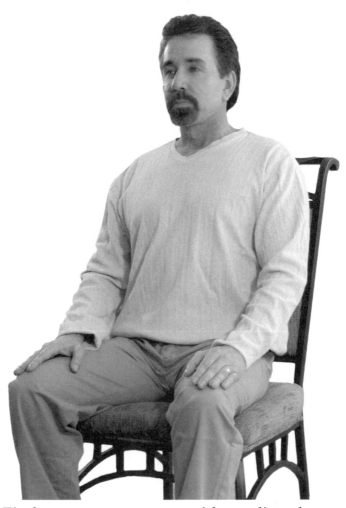

2. Find a room or an area with no disturbances. Make sure there is a comfortable place to sit or lie down. You can lie down, but sitting up is recommended.

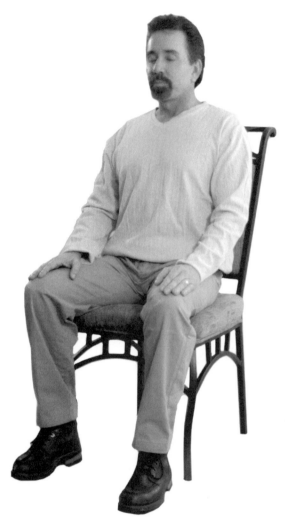

3. Now close your eyes and start the two-minute relaxation technique. Make sure that when you take the breaths, they are as deep as possible without straining yourself.

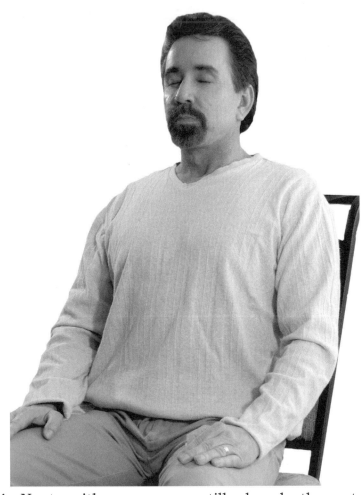

4. Next, with your eyes still closed—they stay closed throughout the entire five-minute process—focus on the food feeling of the food you want to stop eating and its location.

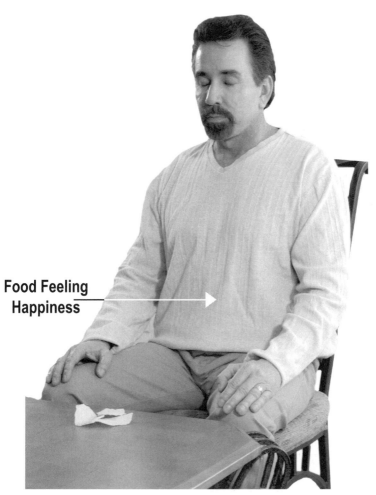

Food Feeling
Happiness

5. As in our example, the food feeling for potato chips is a feeling of happiness and is located in the middle of your stomach. So you would focus on this food feeling (happiness) in the middle of your stomach.

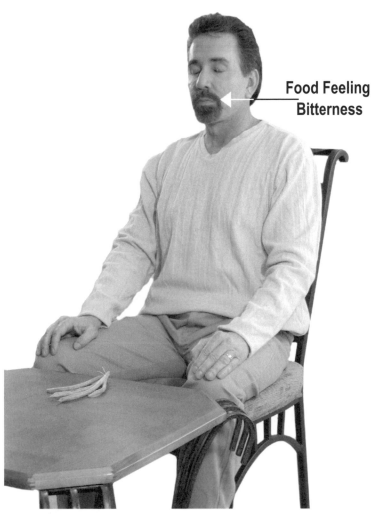

**Food Feeling
Bitterness**

6. After about a minute, clear your mind and quickly shift your focus to the food feeling of the food you dislike and its location in your body. As in our example, the food feeling for green beans (bitterness) is located at the back of your tongue.

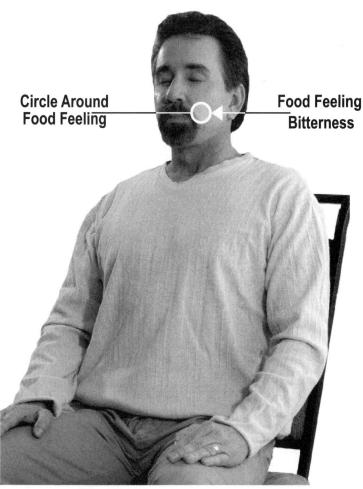

Circle Around Food Feeling   **Food Feeling Bitterness**

7. You are still focused on the food feeling for the food you dislike and its location in your body. Now, mentally draw a circle around the area of this food feeling, enclosing it entirely. Do this visually or non-visually.

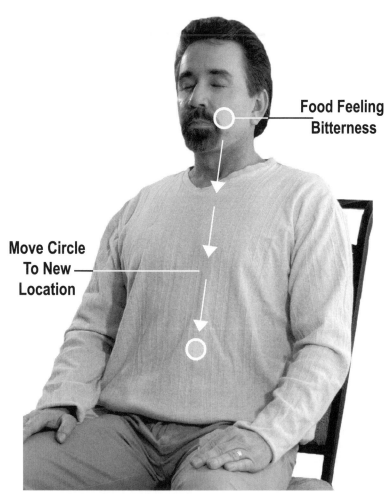

Food Feeling
Bitterness

Move Circle
To New
Location

8. You now have mentally drawn a circle around the food feeling of the food you dislike. Next, move this circle, (visually or non-visually) with the enclosed food feeling to the food feeling location of the junk food. It should only take a few minutes to do this.

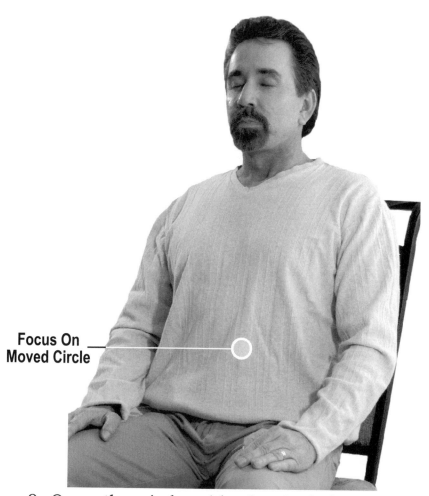

Focus On Moved Circle

9. Once the circle with the food feeling is completely moved to the new location, completely is the key word, continue to focus on the circle and food feeling at this new area for another 30 seconds.

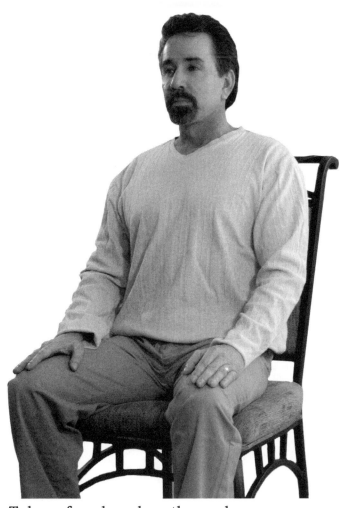

10. Take a few deep breaths and open your eyes.
You are done for the first day.

Food Feelings Program
Next 20 Days

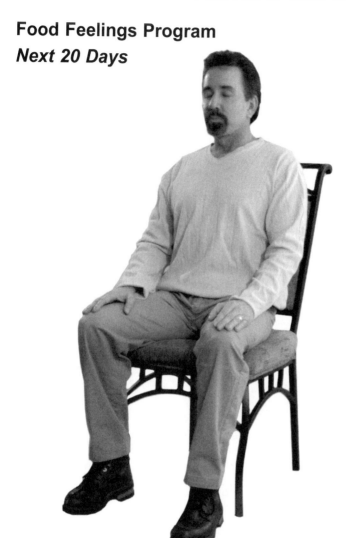

11. Find an area where you will not be disturbed for five minutes. Close your eyes and do the two-minute relaxation technique.

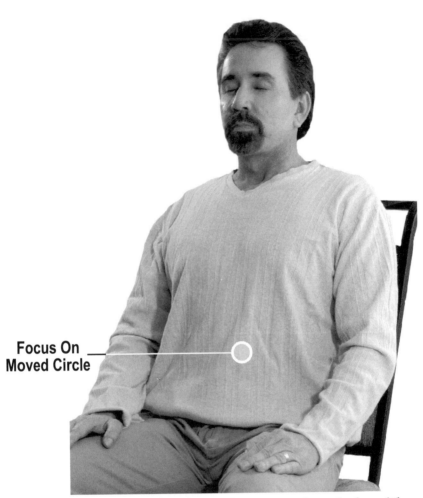

Focus On Moved Circle

12. With eyes still closed, focus on the circle with the food feeling you have previously moved to the new location (example bitterness moved to the middle of the stomach) in your body. Focus intensely on this food feeling in its new area for the next three minutes.

126

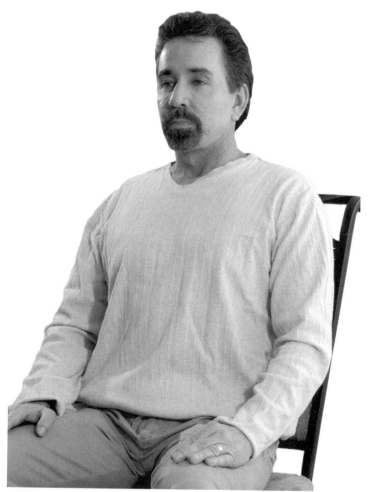

13. After the three minutes, take a deep breath, open your eyes and you are done. Do this five-minute process once a day for the next 20 days.

Index

A

Activated 24

C

Calories 35, 36, 37, 38
Consciously 22, 23, 24
Conscious mind 29, 30

E

Emotions 22
Evoke 22, 25

F

Feelings 21
Food Feelings 16, 17, 21, 22, 24, 49, 60, 61, 72, 92
Food Feelings Program 15, 17, 19, 27, 30, 37, 49, 76, 81, 99

I

Imbed 30, 91
Imbedded 22, 34, 81

L

Linked 91

N

Non-visual 50, 81, 86

R

Reinforcement
  Technique 100
Relaxation Technique 53, 54, 81

S

Sensation 21, 22
Subconscious Mind 28
Subliminally 28

T

Triggered 23, 24

U

Unconscious 24
Unconsciously 23, 30
Unconscious Mind 19, 22, 25, 29, 81

V

Visual 50, 81, 86

W

Weight loss 34, 36

Selected Bibliography

Calm Energy: How People Regulate Mood With Food and Exercise. Robert E. Thayer, Oxford Press.

Conscious Eating. Gabriel Cousens, North Atlantic Books.

Consciousness Explained. Dennett, Daniel Little, Brown & Co.

Doctor's Pocket Calorie, Fat & Carbohydrate Counter, 2003. Allan Borushek, Family Health Pub.

Food and Mood: Second Edition The Complete Guide To Eating Well and Feeling Your Best. Nancy Snyderman, Elizabeth Somer, Owl Books.

Foods That Cause You to Lose Weight: The Negative Calorie Effect. Neal Barnard, Avon.

Frogs Into Princes: Neuro-Linguistic Programming. Richard Bandler and John Grinder, Real People Press.

Hypnotic Realities. Milton Erickson, Ernest Rossi, and Sheila Rossi, Irvington Publishers.

Meta-States: Self-Reflexivity In Human States of Consciousness. Michael L.Hall, E.T. Publications.

Roots of Neuro-Linguistic Programming. Dilts Cupertino, Meta Publications.

The Essential Guide to Nutrition and The Foods We Eat. American Dietetic Association, Harper Resource.

The Everything Calorie Mini Book: Quick and Easy Calorie Counts for All the Foods You Love To Eat. Barbara Ravage, Adams Media Corporation.

The Food and Mood Handbook: Find Relief at Last from Depression, Anxiety, PMS, Cravings and Mood Swings. Amanda Geary, Thorsons.

The Food Bible. Judith Wills, Fireside.

The Mystery of The Mind: A Critical Study of The Consciousness and The Human Brain. Wilder Penfield, Princeton University Press.

The New Whole Foods Encyclopedia: A Comprehensive Resource for Healthy Eating. Rebecca Wood, Penguin USA.

The Quick and Easy Fat Gram & Calorie Counter. Lynn Sonberg, Avon.

Thin Tastes Better Control Your Food Triggers and Lose Weight Without Feeling Deprived. Stephen P. Gullo, Dell.

To buy any of the following Books, Videos, DVDs check with your local bookstore, www.stopeatjunk.com, www.cancerimagery.com, www.healingreiki.com or email bodymindheal@aol.com

VIDEOS & DVDS BY STEVE MURRAY

Preparing Mentally & Emotionally
For Cancer Surgery
A Guided Imagery Program

Preparing Mentally & Emotionally
For Cancer Chemotherapy
A Guided Imagery Program

Preparing Mentally & Emotionally
For Cancer Radiation
A Guided Imagery Program

Preparing Mentally & Emotionally
For Cancer Recovery
A Guided Imagery Program

Dissolving & Destroying Cancer Cells
A Guided Imagery Program

Pain Relief Subliminal Program
Let Your Unconscious Mind Do It!

Fear & Stress Relief Subliminal Program
Let Your Unconscious
Mind Do The Work!

30-Day Subliminal Weight Loss Program
Let Your Unconscious
Mind Do The Work!

30-Day Subliminal Stop Smoking
Program Let Your Unconscious
Mind Do The Work!

Reiki Master Attunement
Become A Reiki Master

Reiki 1st Level Attunement
Give Healing Energy To Yourself
and Others

Reiki Healing Attunement
Heal Emotional-Mental-Physical-
Spiritual Issues

Reiki 2nd Level Attunement
Learn and Use the Reiki Sacred Symbols

BOOKS BY STEVE MURRAY

Cancer Guided Imagery Program
For Radiation, Chemotherapy, Surgery,
And Recovery

Stop Eating Junk!
In 5 Minutes A Day for 21 Days

Reiki The Ultimate Guide
Learn Sacred Symbols and Attunements
Plus Reiki Secrets You Should Know

133

About The Author

Steve Murray is an author and has produced a series of Cancer Guided Imagery video and DVD programs that are used in support groups and hospitals throughout the country. He also has a series of successful DVD and VHS self-help programs on such topics as weight loss, stopping smoking, pain, fear and stress relief.

Steve is a certified Hypnotherapist, and a member of the National League of Medical Hypnotherapists and the National Guild of Hypnotists. He has a private practice and can be contacted through the publisher or directly at:

Email bodymindheal@aol.com or through his web site www.stopeatjunk

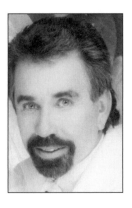

135